The Pink Salt Trick For Weight Loss

Natural Weight Loss Recipes & Mineral-Rich Rituals to Boost Metabolism, Eliminate Bloat, Reset Hormones & Revive Energy—A Pink Salt Healing Guide for Women

Abigail Douglas

Table of Contents

Preface

Why This Book Matters Now—And Why It's Unlike Anything Else You've Tried

If you're holding this book, chances are you're exhausted.

Not just the kind of tired that sleep fixes. But the deeper kind. The kind that comes from battling bloating, unpredictable cravings, stalled weight loss, hormonal chaos, energy crashes, and a sense that your body just isn't listening anymore.

Maybe you've tried every "fat-burning diet," downloaded the free meal plans, cut carbs, counted calories, bought the collagen powder, and promised yourself this time would be different. Maybe you've looked in the mirror and wondered: Why do I feel so off… and what am I missing?

I wrote this book to give you a new answer.

Not another restriction. Not a product pitch. But a ritual—a simple, natural daily practice that taps into your body's original intelligence. A science-backed, soul-soothing method that uses Himalayan pink salt, real hydration, and nervous system support to reset your metabolism, reduce inflammation, rebalance your hormones, and help you feel... like you again.

This is not a diet book. It's a metabolism reset guide rooted in simplicity, minerals, and rhythm—not shame or starvation. Inside, you'll discover:

- **Pink salt recipes** that support fat-burning and hormonal balance
- A **21-day weight loss reset plan** with real meals and rituals that work
- **Debloat drinks, detox soups, and mineral-rich tonics** that soothe your gut and spark your energy
- **Cycle-syncing support** for hormone harmony—without jargon or overwhelm

13

- Daily rituals that help control cravings, boost mood, and rebuild energy—especially for women over 30, 40, and 50

- A completely natural way to **reset your metabolism after burnout**, PMS, menopause, or emotional eating

The results? More energy. Better digestion. Calmer moods. Clothes that fit. A body that feels like home again.

And no—you don't have to give up your coffee. You don't need to buy fancy supplements or force yourself through brutal workouts. What you do need is a clear, repeatable system that honors your biology instead of fighting it. That's what this book offers.

INTRODUCTION

"Why You've Been Tired, Bloated, and Stuck (And Why It's Not Your Fault)"

You're not broken.

You're not lazy.

You're not lacking willpower.

And no—you don't need another diet.

If you've landed here, chances are you've been chasing wellness like it's some slippery, vanishing thing. You've counted calories. You've tried clean eating, keto, smoothies, low-carb-this, low-fat-that. Maybe you even tried to "love your body" while quietly warring with it behind the scenes.

You've felt it, haven't you?

That deep, aching **tiredness** that coffee can't fix.

The mysterious **bloating** that comes out of nowhere,

15

puffing up your belly after a seemingly "healthy" meal.

The cravings that pull you to the pantry after a long day usually for salt or sugar when what you really crave is clarity, relief, balance.

The stubborn **weight gain** that doesn't respond to your efforts, like your body is locked in survival mode.

And the worst part? Everyone tells you it's your fault.

But here's the truth:

It's not your fault.

It's your *body's cry for help*. And no one ever gave you the manual.

The Real Reason You Feel So Off

If you're a woman navigating modern life especially if you're in your 30s, 40s, 50s, or beyond, you are constantly being pulled in a thousand directions. The emails, the expectations, the emotional labor. And while you push through, your body holds the score.

Your hormones don't just control your cycle they influence your metabolism, mood, digestion, cravings, and even how well you sleep. And yet, the very systems designed to protect you often get overwhelmed when you're under chronic stress, eating processed foods, or pushing past your body's natural rhythms.

That exhaustion? It's not in your head—it's in your cells.

That bloat? It's not just food—it's inflammation, mineral imbalances, stress chemistry.

Those cravings? They're not weakness—they're messages.

Your body isn't fighting you—it's **trying to help you**, with the only tools it has left.

My Accidental Discovery (and Why This Book Exists)

A few years ago, I was exactly where you are exhausted,

inflamed, over it. I'd tried everything "healthy." But I was still crashing in the afternoons. Still waking up puffy. Still reaching for comfort food when my brain was foggy and my belly bloated for no good reason.

Then, one morning, I stumbled across a curious conversation online: someone mentioned starting the day with a pinch of **Himalayan pink salt** in warm lemon water. Not for weight loss. Not as a cleanse. But as a simple way to restore electrolytes and support the nervous system.

Skeptical but desperate, I tried it.

And what happened in the next 24 hours changed everything.

That morning, I felt **clearer**—more grounded. My stomach didn't balloon after breakfast. I didn't get hit with the usual 3PM crash. I even slept better that night.

I thought it was a fluke. But I kept going.

Day by day, I started noticing:

- **Fewer cravings** (especially for sugar and chips)
- **Flatter stomach**, especially after meals
- **Better energy**—not wired, but steady and calm
- **More peace** in my body—like I wasn't in a constant fight with myself

And then I started sharing it with friends, clients, and later, a small community of women who all said the same thing:

"Why didn't anyone tell me this sooner?"

So now, I'm telling you.

This Book Is Not a Diet Book

You won't find calorie charts or fat-burning hacks here.

You won't be told to restrict your carbs, suppress your hunger, or punish your body into change.

Instead, you'll be invited into a **ritual**—a gentle rhythm that supports your body with minerals, hydration, and ease. Because pink salt is more than just seasoning. It's a symbol of **what's been missing**:

- **Simplicity** in a world of overwhelm
- **Ritual** in a world of chaos
- **Replenishment** in a world that keeps asking you to give more

Inside this book, you'll learn the truth about metabolism, hormones, energy, and digestion—without the shame or the science degree. You'll find real stories, real recipes, and real shifts that meet you exactly where you are.

Here's What You'll Discover:

- Why your metabolism isn't "slow"—it's **depleted** (and how to wake it up again)
- How pink salt supports your body's **natural hormone rhythms**
- The secret link between **cravings, stress, and salt** (and how to break the cycle)

- The reason your belly feels bloated (and how to **calm your gut** naturally)
- How to use pink salt in **tonics, meals, and body rituals** that feel like self-care, not self-control
- A **21-day plan** that helps you reset without starving, suffering, or starting over (again)

Why Pink Salt?

Himalayan pink salt is packed with trace minerals more than 80 of them that the body needs for everything from hormone function to hydration. It helps **balance electrolytes**, **stimulate digestion**, and **support adrenal function** especially crucial for women under stress.

But more than that, it becomes a powerful *anchor* a physical reminder to stop rushing and start nourishing.

It's not a magic pill.

It's not a quick fix.

It's a return to **body wisdom**—one pinch at a time.

Let's Begin Together

You don't need to be perfect. You don't need a full fridge of superfoods.

You just need a pinch of salt, a moment of quiet, and a willingness to listen to your body again.

This book is your invitation.

To feel lighter.

To feel stronger.

To feel like yourself again—only better.

Welcome to **The Pink Salt Trick**.

Let's get your energy, glow, and balance back—naturally.

CHAPTER 1

The Truth About Metabolism (And Why It's Not Just About Calories)

You've been told for years that weight is a math equation.

Eat less. Move more. Burn more than you consume.

Calories in, calories out. That's the formula, right?

But if you've ever followed every rule—watched what you ate, worked out five days a week, skipped desserts and *still* felt exhausted, bloated, foggy, or stuck on the scale... you've likely whispered to yourself:

"Something's not adding up."

And you're right. Because your metabolism isn't just a calculator.

It's a **conversation. A rhythm. A response**.

It's your body's way of managing energy, processing

nutrients, regulating temperature, and deciding how much to burn or store based on what it senses about your environment.

And for most women, that environment has been chaotic, stressful, undernourished, and out of sync for years.

Your Metabolism Is More Than a Fat-Burning Furnace

Think of metabolism like a symphony. It's not just one solo instrument playing a single note of "burn calories." It's a full orchestra managing:

- How much energy you wake up with
- How your brain stays focused in the afternoon
- How quickly you digest food and eliminate waste
- Whether your body stores fat or uses it for fuel

- If your hormones are signaling "safe to shed" or "must hold on"

When your body feels **safe, supported, and nourished**, it turns on the lights and lets energy flow.

When your body feels **stressed, depleted, or threatened**, it hits the brakes and hoards resources.

This is why you can "do everything right" and still feel like your metabolism is asleep. It's not broken—it's **protecting you**.

The Mineral Deficiency Nobody's Talking About

Let's break this down even further:

Your metabolism can't function without minerals.

Your cells run on **electrical signals**, and those signals are carried by—you guessed it—**electrolytes**. These include sodium, potassium, magnesium, and calcium. If those aren't present in the right amounts, your cells can't create energy efficiently, no matter how clean your diet is.

And what's the #1 mineral women are told to avoid?

Sodium.

Decades of fear around salt have pushed women to cut sodium to the bone, often leading to:

- Low blood pressure
- Dizziness or lightheadedness
- Fatigue after exercise
- Sugar and caffeine cravings
- Trouble concentrating

Meanwhile, real, unrefined pink salt (like Himalayan salt) contains over 80 trace minerals that help **support hydration, digestion, and hormonal function**. It's not the same as table salt. It's a tool of restoration.

Sodium, Potassium & the Adrenal Connection

Now let's talk about a part of your body that's silently influencing everything: your adrenal glands.

These two small glands sit atop your kidneys and are responsible for producing hormones like **cortisol** (stress), **aldosterone** (fluid balance), and **adrenaline** (energy and alertness). When you're constantly under stress (mental or physical), your adrenals pump out cortisol to help you cope.

But here's the kicker:

In order to make those hormones and maintain blood pressure and fluid balance, your adrenals need a delicate balance of **sodium and potassium**.

If sodium is too low (and potassium too high), the body goes into *conservation mode*:

- Fatigue deepens

- Metabolism slows

- Water retention and bloat increase

- You crave sugar, salt, or caffeine like crazy

This is why many women who are eating "healthy," drinking tons of water, and doing all the "right things" still feel inflamed, tired, and out of sync. **They're mineral-depleted.**

And this is where **pink salt comes in like a breath of fresh, mineral-rich air**.

The Morning Metabolism Mix

Let's keep it simple.

You don't need a complicated supplement stack or a $200 cleanse kit.

You need to **wake your cells up gently** and replenish what they've lost overnight.

This one ritual changes everything:

The Morning Metabolism Mix

You'll need:

- 1 glass of warm filtered water (about 12–16 oz)
- Juice of ½ a fresh lemon
- A pinch of high-quality Himalayan pink salt (about ⅛ tsp)
- Optional: a splash of apple cider vinegar or a few drops of raw honey

Instructions:

1. Upon waking, *before coffee*, food, or social media—mix all ingredients in a glass.
2. Sip *slowly*.
3. Breathe deeply. Set an intention. Let your body receive.

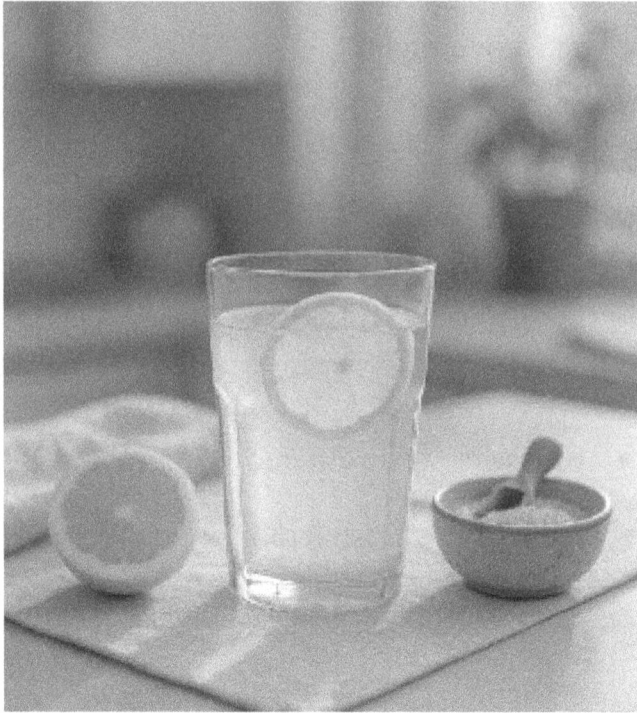

Begin your day with replenishment, not restriction.
Your body will thank you.

What This Ritual Does:

- Replenishes sodium and trace minerals lost during sleep

- Stimulates stomach acid for improved digestion

- Supports adrenal health and hormone balance

- Encourages natural detox through better hydration

- Curbs cravings by satisfying the body's real needs

- Gently wakes up metabolism without a crash

Within just a few mornings, many women report feeling **less bloated**, more energized, and surprisingly **less dependent on caffeine**.

Your metabolism isn't a machine to be forced, it's a system to be **nourished**, **respected**, and **reset**.

What pink salt does is deceptively simple. It doesn't force anything. It doesn't override your biology. It **replenishes what's been missing**, quietly reminding your body:

It's safe to use energy again. It's safe to let go. It's safe to feel good.

In the next chapter, we'll explore how this small act of replenishment has ripple effects throughout your entire hormone system and why most women are unknowingly operating in a deficit that pink salt can help close.

Ready to get your rhythm back?

Let's keep going.

CHAPTER 2

Hormones Out of Whack? Here's What Pink Salt Really Does

Have you ever stood in front of the mirror and thought,

"I don't even recognize this body anymore"?

The stubborn belly bloat that won't go away, no matter how "clean" you eat.

The unpredictable mood swings that make you feel like a stranger to yourself.

The energy crashes, the sleep issues, the unexplainable weight gain…

It's easy to blame yourself.

And that's what the wellness world often trains us to do.

But what if I told you:

Your body isn't failing. It's protecting you.

And what looks like a breakdown… is actually a response.

Modern Stress Is Rewiring Your Hormones

Let's be real: modern life is *relentless*.

You're expected to juggle family, work, emotional labor, and self-care without ever letting the ball drop. And while you're holding it all together on the outside, your **hormones** are carrying the invisible cost.

The truth is, your body was never designed to live in a state of constant urgency.

And when stress is chronic whether it's from deadlines, lack of sleep, blood sugar swings, or unresolved emotions—your hormones don't just get "out of balance." They **shift into survival mode**.

Here's what that looks like…

Cortisol: Your Body's Emergency Responder

Cortisol is your stress hormone. It's not the villain, it's your built-in alarm system. It raises your blood sugar to give you energy, increases alertness, and temporarily suppresses non-essential systems like digestion and reproduction.

But when cortisol is elevated *all* the time?

- Your metabolism slows down
- You crave sugar, salt, and caffeine
- Your sleep becomes shallow or restless
- Your belly stores fat to "protect your organs"
- You feel anxious, wired, and eventually... *burned out*

And that's where **adrenal fatigue** begins, not as a sudden crash, but as a slow depletion.

Estrogen Dominance & Hormonal Confusion

Meanwhile, for women especially, this stress loop creates a **cascade of hormonal confusion**.

Many experience something called **estrogen dominance**—a state where estrogen levels are high *relative* to progesterone, even if both are technically "normal." This can lead to:

- PMS and bloating
- Breast tenderness
- Weight gain around the hips and midsection
- Anxiety and mood swings
- Heavy or irregular periods

Combine this with low magnesium, poor hydration, and a fast-paced lifestyle… and you get a hormonal symphony that's completely out of tune.

So how does pink salt play into all of this?

Pink Salt: The Mineral Support Your Hormones Are Begging For

Your body doesn't run on willpower, it runs on *minerals*.

And here's the truth most people don't know:

Stress burns through minerals at a rapid rate.

The more cortisol your body produces, the more it depletes:

- **Sodium**
- **Potassium**
- **Magnesium**
- **Calcium**

These minerals regulate fluid balance, nerve signaling, muscle contraction, digestion, and yes—**hormone production and detoxification**.

What makes **Himalayan pink salt** so powerful isn't just that it's natural. It's because it contains over 84 trace minerals, including the ones most women are unknowingly lacking.

How Trace Minerals Support Hormonal Balance

Let's break it down simply:

- **Sodium & Potassium** – help regulate adrenal hormones like aldosterone and cortisol
- **Magnesium** – supports progesterone levels and calms the nervous system
- **Calcium** – crucial for estrogen metabolism and PMS symptom relief
- **Zinc & Selenium** – key players in thyroid hormone conversion and reproductive health

- **Iodine (trace amounts)** – supports thyroid gland function

By gently reintroducing these minerals daily, you're giving your endocrine system the building blocks it needs to **come back into rhythm**.

Pink salt doesn't override your hormones, it **reminds them how to function harmoniously**.

Morning & Evening Hormone Reset Rituals

To support your hormones holistically, the key is to create **calming, mineral-rich rituals** that anchor your nervous system and rehydrate your cells.

Here are two simple daily practices that work together like magic:

Morning Ritual – The Hormone Harmony Elixir

Start your day with:

- 12–16 oz of warm filtered water

- Juice of ½ lemon

- ⅛ tsp of Himalayan pink salt

- Optional: a splash of unsweetened cranberry juice (liver & estrogen support)

This blend wakes up digestion, hydrates cells, and helps flush excess estrogen through liver pathways.

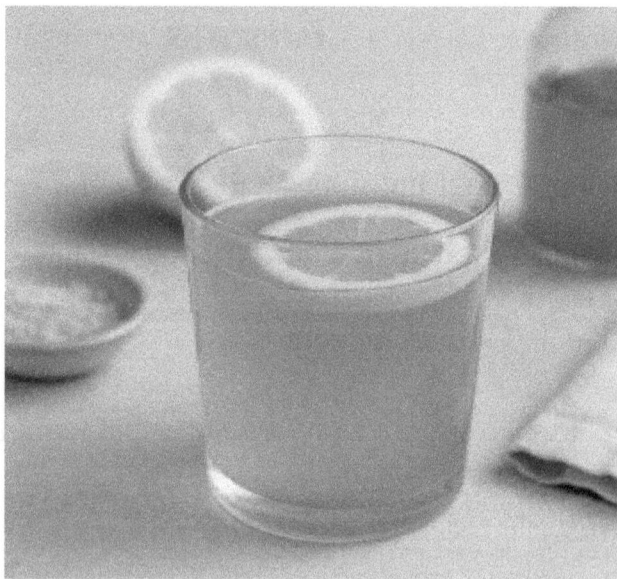

Take a deep breath. Sip it slowly. Let your body receive.

Evening Ritual – The Salted Sleep Soothe

Before bed, try this:

- 1 cup of warm chamomile or ginger tea

- Add a pinch of pink salt

- Optional: 1 tsp raw honey for added calm and blood sugar stabilization

This signals to your nervous system:

"It's safe to rest now."

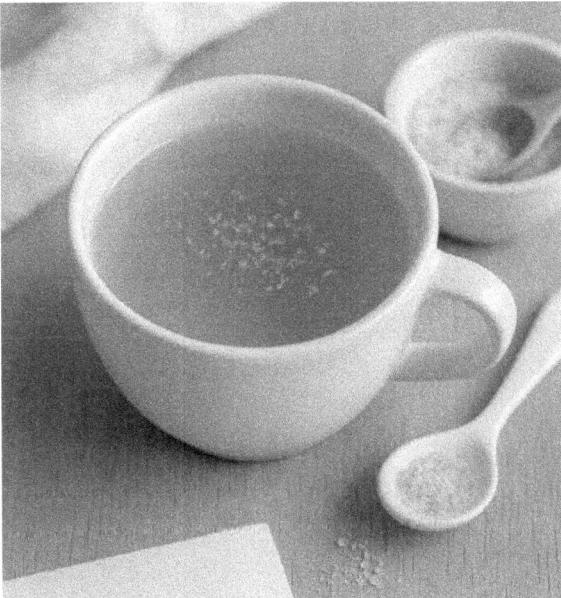

No alarms. No stress. Just healing.

Why These Tiny Changes Matter More Than You Think

The beauty of this ritual isn't just in what it contains—it's in what it represents.

Every time you mix a glass of pink salt water, you're choosing:

- Restoration over restriction
- Replenishment over punishment
- Ritual over chaos

You're telling your hormones, your cells, and your nervous system:

"I've got you."

And in response, your body says:

"Okay. Let's heal."

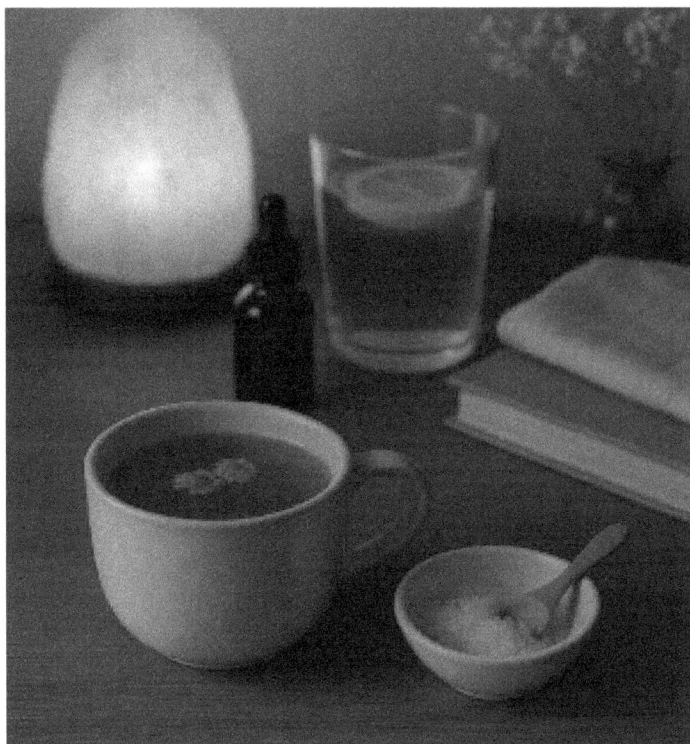

Your body isn't broken, it's just asking to be replenished. Create space for calm. Let the healing begin.

Now that you understand how pink salt supports internal harmony, let's talk about something women wrestle with daily—cravings, stress eating, and emotional hunger.

CHAPTER 3

Cravings, Stress & Salt: The Connection You've Never Heard

You swore you weren't going to snack tonight.

You had a good dinner. You're not technically hungry. But somehow... there you are, standing in the pantry at 9:03 p.m., staring down the chocolate, the chips, or that half-eaten bag of trail mix like it's calling your name.

You're not alone.

Millions of women experience the exact same cycle every day.

But here's the truth that no one ever tells you:

It's not about willpower.

It's not about discipline, or how "bad" you were during the day.

Cravings especially those for salt, sugar, and carbs are not failures.

They are messages.

And the body is whispering something important underneath every urge.

Decoding Cravings, Snacking & Emotional Eating

Let's talk about the most misunderstood symptoms in the world of women's health:

- Sugar cravings
- Carb addiction
- Late-night snacking
- "Emotional" hunger

These are so often labeled as weaknesses, when in truth, they are signals. Signals that the body is:

- **Under-fueled**
- **Mineral-depleted**
- **Emotionally frayed**
- **Operating under stress chemistry** rather than safety

When your body senses a threat whether it's physical (like skipping meals), emotional (stress or anxiety), or energetic (overwork, under-sleep) it shifts gears.

And one of the first things it does?

Demand fast, comforting fuel.

Usually in the form of sweet or salty carbs.

Because sugar = quick glucose

And salt = a fast hit of missing minerals

Your brain doesn't want to sabotage you. It wants to **save you**.

The Science: Stress Depletes Sodium—and That Worsens Cravings

When you're under chronic stress, your adrenal glands pump out cortisol to keep you alert, help manage blood sugar, and stabilize blood pressure.

But cortisol doesn't work alone. It relies heavily on **aldosterone**, a hormone that regulates **sodium retention** and **fluid balance**.

Here's where it gets fascinating:

- When aldosterone levels drop (as they often do in chronic stress or adrenal fatigue), the body **excretes too much sodium** through urine.
- As sodium levels fall, the body begins to **crave** salty or sweet foods as a survival mechanism.

- Low sodium also makes it hard for cells to retain water, causing **dehydration**, dizziness, fatigue, and more cravings.

So the next time you're craving chips at night, consider this:

It might not be about your emotions.

It might be your *body screaming for salt*.

Enter: The 3PM Craving Calm Salt Sip

There's a window in the day usually around 2:30 to 4:00 p.m. where everything catches up to you.

Your focus dips.

Your patience wears thin.

Your blood sugar drops.

And cravings hit like clockwork.

Instead of reaching for sugar or caffeine, try this reset ritual:

The 3PM Craving Calm Salt Sip

Ingredients:

- 12 oz warm or room-temperature filtered water
- 1 tablespoon apple cider vinegar (with the mother)
- ⅛ teaspoon Himalayan pink salt
- A pinch of cinnamon
- Optional: a drop of raw honey or a cinnamon stick to stir

Instructions:

1. Mix all ingredients in a glass or mug.
2. Sip slowly, breathing deeply between sips.
3. Let your nervous system and mineral balance recalibrate.

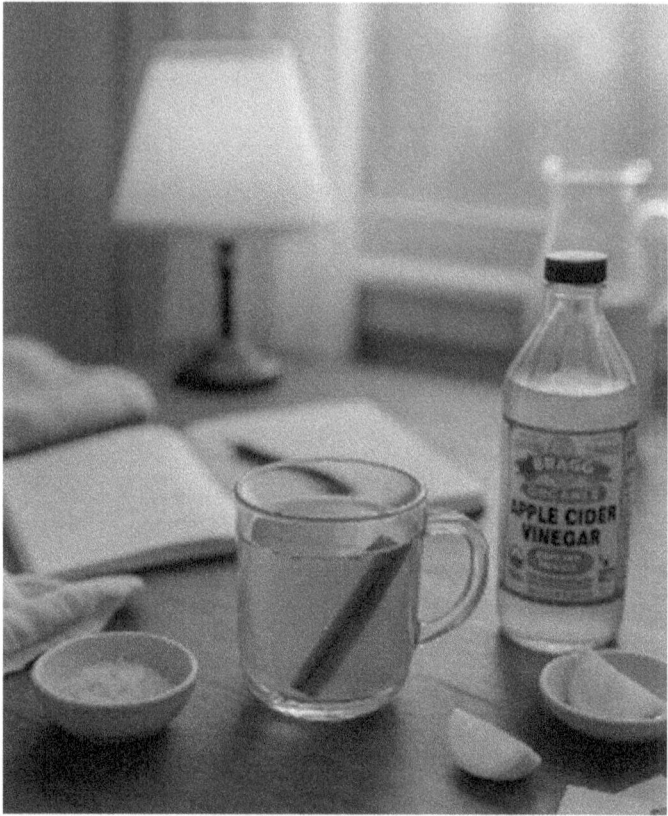

Cravings don't mean you've failed. They mean your body is asking to be nourished. Pause. Sip. Replenish

Why It Works:

- **Apple cider** vinegar stabilizes blood sugar
- **Pink salt** replenishes minerals lost to stress

- **Cinnamon** helps regulate insulin and gives a natural sweet aroma

- **Warm water** soothes digestion and signals safety

This drink doesn't just "distract" you from cravings, it satisfies the **root cause**: mineral deficiency, blood sugar imbalance, and emotional overwhelm.

Emotional Awareness Tool: "The Craving Is a Messenger"

Let's add one more layer to this ritual—emotional awareness.

When a craving shows up, instead of judging it, ask:

- What am I *really* needing right now?

- Am I tired, anxious, overstimulated, or undernourished?

- Is this hunger for food—or for peace, relief, connection?

Cravings are not enemies. They are invitations.

Not to restrict. But to *replenish*.

Not to shame yourself. But to listen deeper.

Sometimes, a pinch of salt and five minutes of stillness can bring you back to center faster than any snack ever could.

Cravings Aren't the Problem— They're the Clue

In a world that teaches us to control and criticize our bodies, learning to interpret cravings is revolutionary.

They are not weaknesses.

They are the **voice of your body asking to be fed, held, and heard**.

And sometimes, that voice says:

"I don't need sugar. I need support."

"I don't need punishment. I need peace."

"I don't need less food. I need more minerals."

With the pink salt ritual, you're not silencing your cravings.

You're answering them with kindness—and biochemical truth.

You've learned how cravings are linked to your stress, minerals, and emotional state. You've gained a tool to calm that crash and reconnect with your body's wisdom.

Now, in the next chapter, we'll explore the one thing that affects every woman, often silently:

Bloat.

And how pink salt plays a surprisingly powerful role in supporting digestion, gut flow, and beating the belly bulge—naturally.

Let's go there next.

CHAPTER 4

Bloat Be Gone: The Digestion Reset Your Gut Will Love

Let's talk about a silent struggle that almost every woman knows intimately—but rarely talks about outside whispered complaints in leggings:

Bloating.

It sneaks up out of nowhere.

You eat something healthy, but feel swollen like a balloon.

Your jeans fit in the morning, but by 2PM, you're reaching for elastic waistbands.

You feel full, tight, puffy—even if the scale hasn't moved.

And it doesn't just affect how you look. It affects how you feel.

Bloated = uncomfortable.

Bloated = tired, sluggish, self-conscious, distracted.

But here's what the wellness world doesn't often tell you:

Bloating isn't random. It's a signal.

A cue that your digestion needs support—not more fiber or detox pills.

And one of the most surprising (and simple) tools to relieve it?

A pinch of pink salt.

What Is Bloat *Really*?

Bloat isn't always about food volume or calories. It's about how your body processes, breaks down, and moves what you eat.

There are 3 common forms of bloating:

1. **Fluid Retention:** Caused by poor mineral balance, hormone shifts, or dehydration

2. **Inflammation:** Triggered by food sensitivities, stress, or imbalanced gut flora

3. **Slowed Motility:** When digestion is sluggish and food sits too long in the gut

All three create that full, heavy, uncomfortable feeling. But all three also point back to the same root system:

Your digestive fire.

Why Pink Salt Is a Digestion Hero

Digestion begins before you even swallow. It starts with your brain signaling your stomach to **produce hydrochloric acid (HCl),** the acid needed to break down protein, absorb nutrients, and kill pathogens.

And guess what plays a huge role in triggering that stomach acid?

Sodium chloride—aka, salt.

But not just any salt.

Himalayan pink salt provides natural sodium plus 80+ trace minerals that support the entire digestive cascade.

Here's what pink salt can help with:

- Stimulates **stomach acid production** for smoother digestion
- Activates **bile release** from the liver to emulsify fats
- Aids **enzyme function** in the pancreas
- Helps balance gut **pH levels** to reduce gas and fermentation
- Enhances **electrolyte flow** to support intestinal motility

This means food gets broken down better, moves more efficiently through your system, and **bloating naturally fades**.

The Pink Salt Debloat Tonic

If you've ever felt like your belly "puffs up" out of nowhere, try this. It's fast. It's soothing. And it works.

Pink Salt Debloat Tonic

Ingredients:

- 1 cup warm water
- Juice of ½ fresh lemon
- ⅛ tsp Himalayan pink salt
- ½ tsp grated fresh ginger (or a slice)
- ¼ tsp ground fennel seeds (or steep 1 tsp whole seeds in hot water)

Instructions:

1. Add all ingredients to a mug.
2. Steep 5–10 minutes, then sip slowly before or after meals.

3. For extra support, add a drop of raw honey or drink while gently massaging your belly clockwise.

Why These Ingredients Work:

- **Lemon** stimulates bile and enzyme production
- **Ginger** warms the gut and improves motility
- **Fennel** relieves gas, calms the intestines, and reduces cramping
- **Pink salt** wakes up the digestive process with minerals and sodium

Use this tonic anytime you feel bloated, or make it part of your daily pre-lunch ritual.

The Bedtime Bloat-Relief Ritual

Digestion doesn't stop when you sleep. In fact, your body does some of its deepest gut healing overnight. If your belly feels backed up, slow, or heavy before bed, try this calming support:

Salted Warm Water Sleep Soothe

Ingredients:

- 8 oz warm filtered water
- A pinch of Himalayan pink salt
- Optional: Chamomile or peppermint tea bag
- Optional: ½ tsp honey (for blood sugar balance)

Instructions:

1. Mix the salt into the warm water (or herbal tea).
2. Sip slowly about 30–60 minutes before bed.
3. Breathe deeply. Rub your belly. Let your body reset.

This helps ease constipation, reduce fluid retention, and stimulate mild bile flow for smoother elimination by morning.

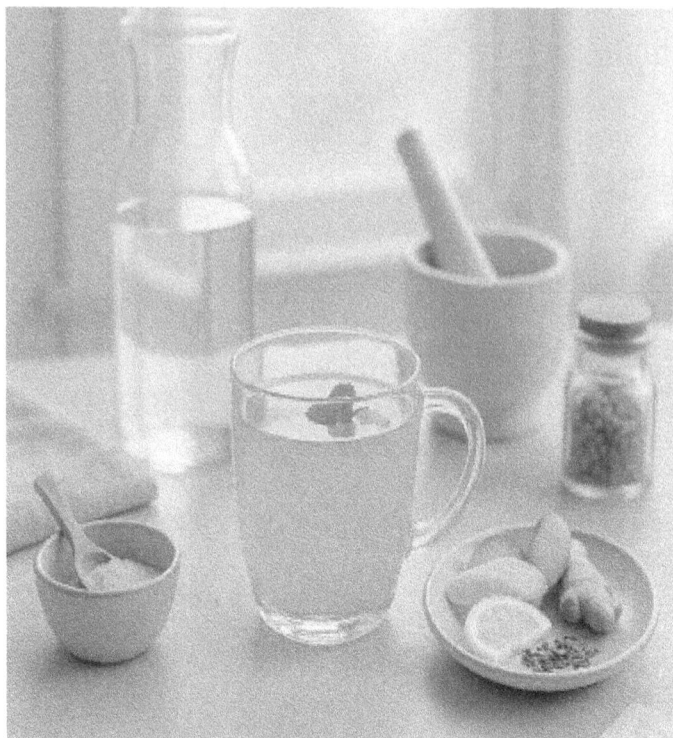

You don't need to shrink body – just help it flow. Bloat isn't failure. It's a signal for support.

Belly Bloat Isn't Just a Food Problem—It's a Flow Problem

The world will tell you to "cut carbs" or "eat cleaner." But most women don't need less food, they need **better**

digestion.

You need warmth. Movement. Acid. Enzymes. Mineral balance.

You need a nervous system that believes, "It's safe to rest. It's safe to digest."

And the ritual of sipping salt-infused herbal drinks?

It's a message to your body:

"I'm not going to fight you anymore. I'm going to work with you."

That's where healing begins. That's when bloat ends.

In the next chapter, we'll move from digestion to energy. Because once the bloat is gone, the next thing most women crave is… vitality. The kind that doesn't rely on caffeine or adrenaline. The kind that pink salt quietly helps you reclaim.

Let's talk about that next.

CHAPTER 5

Pink Salt & Natural Energy: No More Midday Slumps

There's a moment around midday when it hits you—like a wall.

Your eyes glaze over. Your head feels heavy. You yawn without warning.

And your body whispers the same desperate question it whispered yesterday:

"Where did my energy go?"

It doesn't matter if you had a full night's sleep. Or if you started the day strong.

That 2PM–4PM window seems to *steal your spark* every time.

So you reach for something. Coffee. Chocolate. A second

lunch. Anything to get your brain back online. But the boost doesn't last. It never does.

Because what your body *really* needs… isn't caffeine.

It's **minerals.**

It's Not Just Dehydration. It's Cellular Depletion.

We've all been told to "drink more water" to fight fatigue. And yes, water matters. But here's what most health advice gets wrong:

Water without minerals ≠ hydration.

In fact, drinking too much plain water especially when you're already mineral-deficient can actually make fatigue worse by flushing out precious electrolytes.

Your cells need **sodium, potassium, magnesium, calcium** and other trace minerals to move water into the cells where it's useful.

Without those minerals?

- Water passes right through you

- You feel bloated but thirsty

- Your brain stays foggy

- Your muscles stay tense

- Your energy stays flat

In other words: **You're not tired, you're *mineral-depleted*.**

Sodium = The Spark of Energy

Let's zoom in on one essential mineral: sodium.

Sodium gets a bad rap because of processed food and blood pressure myths, but here's the truth:

You cannot create cellular energy (ATP) without sodium.

Sodium:

- Regulates **nerve impulses** and **muscle contraction**

- Supports **adrenal health** and cortisol balance

- Helps deliver **glucose** into your cells for fuel

- Balances **fluid inside and outside your cells**

- Works with potassium and magnesium to power the **mitochondria**—your energy factories

So when you feel "burnt out," what you often need isn't motivation or more protein.

You need **electrolyte-supported hydration** and pink salt is your simplest solution.

The Salt-Infused Hydration Ritual

This is one of the easiest (and most transformative) changes you can make:

Daily Energy Bottle Ritual

Ingredients:

- 24 oz filtered water

- ⅛ tsp Himalayan pink salt

- Squeeze of fresh lemon or lime

- Optional: 1 tsp coconut water or a few drops of trace mineral drops

- Optional: sprig of mint or a few cucumber slices

Instructions:

1. Mix ingredients in a glass or stainless steel water bottle.

2. Sip throughout the morning (or afternoon) to avoid crashes.

3. Make this your go-to hydration instead of plain water or sugary drinks.

Why It Works:

- Supports electrolyte balance and intracellular hydration

- Wakes up your cells without caffeine

- Balances blood sugar and prevents the dreaded afternoon slump
- Prevents brain fog, tension headaches, and that "wired but tired" feeling

Many women report that after just 3–4 days of this practice, they **naturally stop craving coffee, soda, or sweets in the afternoon**. Their body stops begging for energy because it finally has enough.

Bonus: Pink Salt + Magnesium Soaks for Recovery & Deep Sleep

If your energy dips come with muscle soreness, tight shoulders, or restless sleep, this nighttime ritual is your reset button.

Evening Mineral Bath for Restoration

Ingredients:

- 1 cup Epsom salt (magnesium sulfate)

- ¼ cup Himalayan pink salt

- Optional: a few drops of lavender or eucalyptus essential oil

- Optional: sliced lemon or fresh herbs in the water for sensory calm

Instructions:

1. Run a warm bath. Add salts and optional oils.

2. Soak for 20–30 minutes while breathing deeply.

3. Hydrate before and after with a pinch of pink salt in warm water.

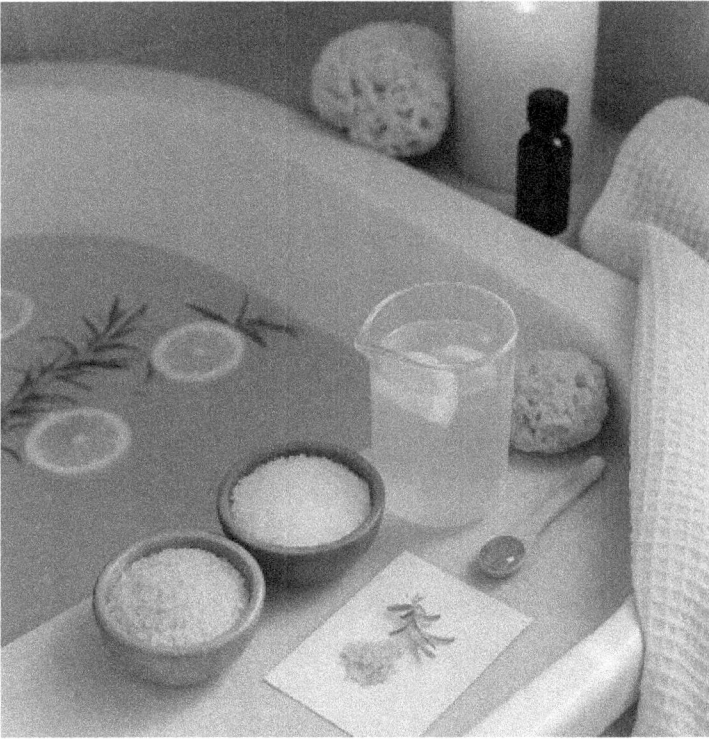

Evening Mineral Bath

This helps:

- Replenish minerals lost from stress or workouts

- Soothe sore muscles and release tension

- Calm the nervous system and support melatonin production

- Deepen sleep quality, which further restores natural energy the next day

Energy Is Not Just a Physical Thing—It's a Signal of Safety

Your body won't give you full energy if it thinks it's unsafe.

Low mineral levels = stress

Stress = conservation mode

Conservation mode = less energy, more cravings, more inflammation

When you restore minerals like pink salt throughout the day, you're not just hydrating.

You're sending a message:

"It's okay to wake up now. You're safe."

And that's when your natural energy returns—not from stimulation, but from true replenishment.

Now that your energy is on the rise, let's talk about how it shows up in your body—through glow, calm, clarity, and hormonal rhythm. In the next chapter, you'll learn how to use pink salt to enhance hormone balance even further, including tips for syncing with your cycle and supporting long-term vibrancy.

CHAPTER 6

The Ritual Reset: How to Rewire Your Body in 21 Days

There's a quiet revolution that begins the moment you stop punishing your body and start supporting it. No scales. No tracking apps. No exhausting willpower games. Just you, a glass of mineral-rich pink salt water, and a decision to come home to yourself.

This chapter is not another plan to follow, it's a path back to rhythm. A chance to exhale the chaos and rebuild trust with your body. And it starts with a daily ritual so simple it might feel too easy to matter… until it changes everything.

Why Simplicity Creates Momentum

We often believe that transformation requires intensity. But what rewires us isn't intensity—it's consistency. Especially for women, whose nervous systems crave safety and stability to release weight, reset hormones, and digest properly.

Your body doesn't need another shock. It needs a signal. A simple, repeatable act of support. That's what the Pink Salt Ritual is: a daily nudge that tells your system, "You're safe now. You can let go."

This chapter will guide you through a three-week reset that gently reshapes your metabolism, digestion, energy, and emotional relationship with food. It's not about perfection. It's about pattern.

The Power of Rituals for Nervous System Healing

Science now confirms what ancient traditions have always known: **ritual is medicine.**

When your nervous system is in fight-or-flight, your body holds onto fat, craves quick energy (sugar), and shuts down digestion. But when you create tiny daily rituals especially ones involving hydration, minerals, breath, or calm, your nervous system shifts from chaos to calm.

In this safe state, your body starts:

- Releasing stored water and inflammation
- Rebalancing hormones
- Calming cravings and blood sugar spikes
- Increasing mitochondrial (cellular energy) function

This is what the Pink Salt Reset is designed to do—**not through effort, but through rhythm.**

How to Use This Chapter

Each week below builds on the last. You'll find:

- A weekly theme (what you're focusing on)
- Simple daily salt-based rituals
- A printable blueprint/checklist you can use as a daily companion

Go gently. Let your body catch up to your intention. And when you miss a day? Just come back. Rituals don't punish—they welcome.

WEEK 1: Calm the Cravings

Theme: Reduce the urge to binge, snack late at night, or reach for sugar when stressed.

What's Happening in Your Body:

- Mineral depletion is being replenished
- Sodium and potassium levels begin balancing
- Blood sugar starts to stabilize
- Adrenal glands are getting support

Daily Rituals:

- **Morning Metabolism Mix:** 1 glass warm water + ½ lemon + pinch of pink salt
  (Sip slowly and set an intention)

- **3PM Craving Calm Sip:** Water + splash of apple cider vinegar + cinnamon + pink salt
  (Drink when the urge to snack strikes)

- **Evening Salt Soak (2–3x/week):** Warm bath + 1 cup Epsom salt + 1 tbsp pink salt

  (Optional drops of lavender or magnesium oil)

Reminder: Cravings are messengers, not enemies. When you hydrate and remineralize, cravings often disappear naturally.

WEEK 2: Reset Digestion

Theme: Relieve bloat, improve motility, reduce inflammation, and support nutrient absorption.

What's Happening in Your Body:

- Hydrochloric acid production increases (essential for digestion)
- Gut motility speeds up
- Bloating decreases

- Your gut-brain axis begins to relax

Daily Rituals:

- **Debloat Tonic Before Meals:** Warm water + pink salt + grated ginger + lemon + fennel

  (Take 15 mins before largest meal)

- **Salted Herbal Digestive Tea:** Chamomile or peppermint tea + pinch of salt

  (Especially soothing in the evening)

- **5-Minute Gut Walk:** After meals, gently walk or stretch to support digestion

  (Movement boosts lymph flow and GI motility)

Reminder: Bloat is not fat. It's a signal your digestion is overwhelmed. Ritual helps your gut feel safe enough to release.

WEEK 3: Balance Energy &

Hormones

Theme: Stabilize mood, reduce PMS symptoms, lift brain fog, and support sustainable energy.

What's Happening in Your Body:

- Cortisol begins to level out
- Estrogen and progesterone rebalance
- Blood sugar and energy spikes reduce
- Sleep and mental clarity improve

Daily Rituals:

- **Salt-Infused Hydration Bottle:** Water + lemon slices + mint + pinch of salt

  (Keep on desk or carry throughout the day)

- **Bedtime Hormone Reboot:** Warm water + pink salt + magnesium powder (optional)

(Calms nervous system and supports hormone detox overnight)

- **Sunlight + Salt Moment:** Spend 5–10 minutes in morning sun with a glass of salted lemon water (Reboots your circadian rhythm and cortisol curve)

Reminder: You're not lazy or "unmotivated." Your energy is tied to your minerals and hormones. Ritual restores flow.

The 21-Day Pink Salt Ritual Blueprint

Each day you'll check off:

- Morning Metabolism Mix
- Midday Salt Sip or Digestive Tonic
- Evening Ritual (Tea, Soak, or Hormone Reboot)
- A moment of mindfulness or journaling

Don't worry if you miss one. The ritual isn't a rule—it's a rhythm. Keep flowing forward.h day, you'll check off:

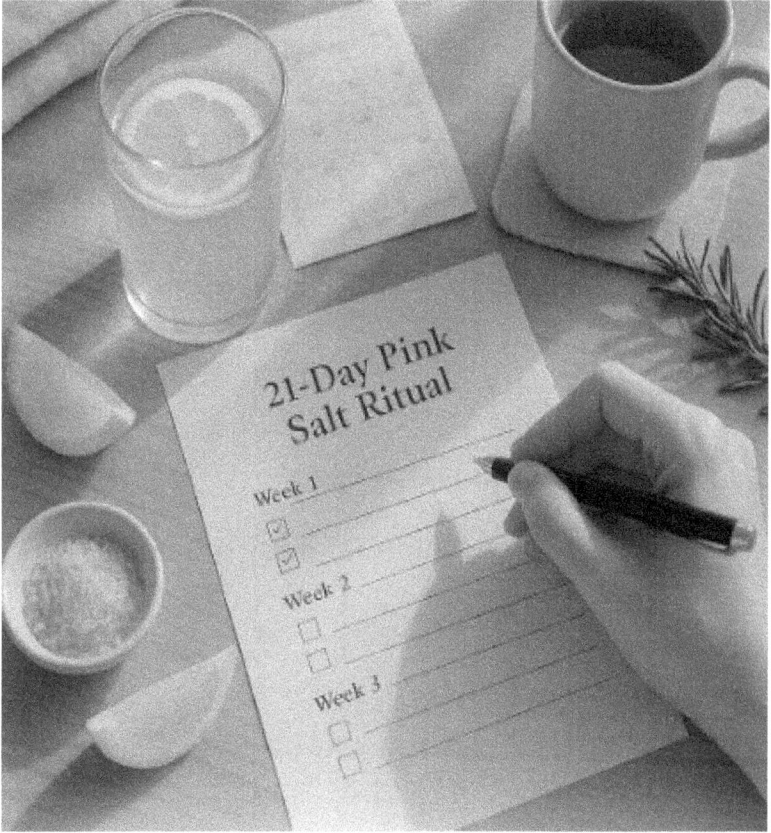

Rituals rewire your body faster than rules. One calm sip. One clear intention

What to Expect by Day 21

Most readers report:

- A reduction in cravings

- Visibly less bloating and puffiness

- Improved energy and digestion

- Less PMS or hormonal mood swings

- A deepened sense of calm and clarity

And perhaps most importantly: they no longer feel afraid of food or their body.

This Is the Reset You Deserve

You were never broken. Your body has simply been overworked, undernourished, and begging for rhythm. These pink salt rituals aren't magic—but your consistency is.

What you practice, your body remembers. And in just 21 days, you'll begin to feel that remembrance deep in your bones:

- ✓ Nourishment over punishment
- ✓ Rhythm over restriction
- ✓ Energy over exhaustion

This isn't a quick fix. It's a quiet return to balance.

Welcome home.

CHAPTER 7

Salt in the Kitchen: Everyday Recipes That Heal (and Taste Good)

Let's set the record straight: food is not your enemy and salt, when chosen wisely, can be one of your greatest healing allies.

This chapter isn't about following strict calorie counts or depriving yourself of flavor. It's about embracing the truth that your kitchen is the most powerful pharmacy in the world. With a few sprinkles of pink salt, some mineral-rich ingredients, and intentional pairings, you can create meals that *nourish, reset*, and *satisfy* all while supporting your metabolism, digestion, and hormonal flow.

And the best part? These recipes are ridiculously doable. No five-hour cooking marathons. No ingredients you can't pronounce. Just simple, healing, crave-worthy dishes you'll return to again and again.

Why Pink Salt Belongs in Every Meal

Pink Himalayan salt is more than just pretty—it's functionally supportive of the systems your body leans on most when trying to regulate weight, energy, and mood. Its naturally occurring trace minerals (like magnesium, calcium, potassium, and iron) help balance electrolytes, support adrenal health, and ignite digestive enzymes.

When used correctly in food, not in excess or in fake "low-sodium" alternatives it helps regulate hydration, calm inflammation, and reduce bloat.

This chapter is your real-life salt-powered toolkit.

Morning Tonics & Mineral Waters

Wake your system with hydration that matters.

- **The Metabolism Morning Mix** (Warm lemon, pink salt, and trace minerals)
- **Cucumber-Mint Mineral Water**
- **Apple Cider & Salt Electrolyte Shot**
- **Cranberry Hormone Flush Tonic**
- **Celtic Calm Elixir** (Pink salt, ginger, and basil water infusion)

Each drink is designed to kickstart digestion, reduce cravings, and restore adrenal resilience.

Debloat Smoothies & Healing Broths

Blends that are gentle, energizing, and gut-soothing.

- **The Anti-Bloat Green Glow Smoothie** (Fennel, mint, pineapple, and salt)

- **Salted Ginger-Banana Calm Shake**

- **Golden Broth with Turmeric & Salted Bone Base**

- **Evening Bloat-Relief Soup** (Celery, parsley, lemon, and salt)

- **Salted Coconut Gut-Healing Smoothie**

Detox Soups with a Pink Salt Kick

Salt enhances digestion and circulation—especially in warm, nutrient-dense soups.

- **Hormone Harmony Carrot-Ginger Soup**

- **Pink Salt & Seaweed Metabolism Stew**

- **Chickpea & Kale Anti-Craving Soup**

- **Detox Miso with Garlic & Salted Nori**

- **Spiced Cabbage Cleanse Broth**

Snacks That Stop Cravings

Snack smart, not less. Craving control starts with mineral balance.

- **Salted Tahini-Cacao Energy Balls**
- **Cucumber + Pink Salt + Lemon Snack Plate**
- **Salt & Vinegar Roasted Chickpeas**
- **Avocado Slices with Salted Lime Dust**
- **Pink Salt Chia Bites with Cinnamon**

These are the "pause-and-replenish" moments that replace stress eating with mineral satisfaction.

Dinner Recipes to Reduce Inflammation

Healing doesn't require restriction—just intention.

- **Salted Lemon Chicken with Roasted Veggies**
- **Spiced Lentils with Salt & Coconut Yogurt Drizzle**
- **Sweet Potato Bowls with Salted Tahini Dressing**
- **Pink Salt Herb-Rubbed Salmon**
- **Anti-Bloat Grain-Free Stir Fry with Pink Salt and Ginger**

These dinner options are deeply nourishing and free from the inflammatory ingredients that spike cortisol, cravings, and blood sugar.

Bonus: Salt Beauty Scrubs & Soaks

Healing isn't just about what goes in it's about what relaxes, grounds, and restores you from the outside in.

- **Glow & Flow Pink Salt Body Scrub (Coconut oil, citrus peel, pink salt)**

- **Anti-Bloat Foot Soak (Epsom + Pink Salt + Peppermint)**

- **Adrenal Recovery Bath Soak (Lavender, pink salt, and magnesium flakes)**

Use these as weekly rituals to calm inflammation, improve circulation, and signal safety to your nervous system.

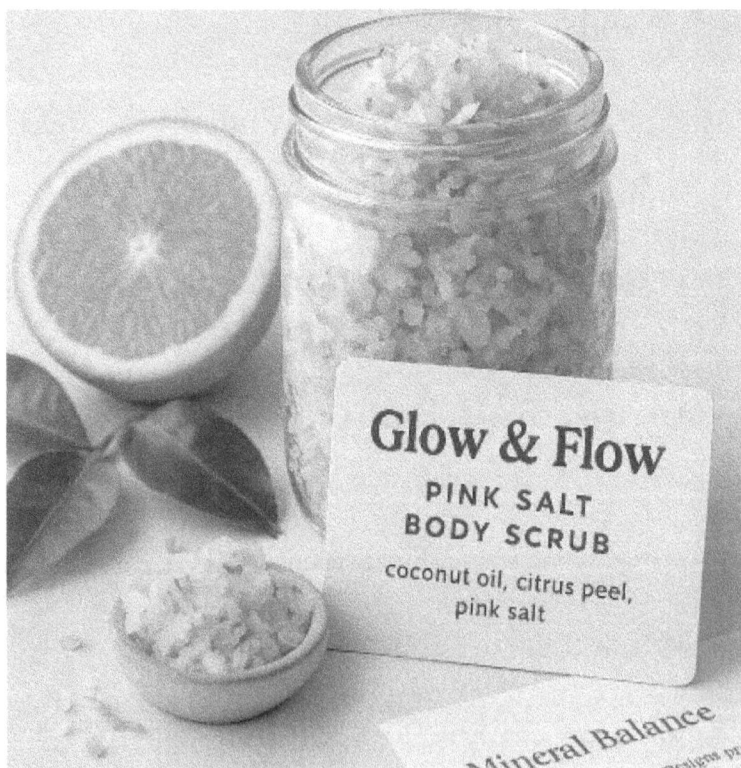

Mineral Balance Bath Soak

What Makes These Recipes Work?

They're based on three core principles:

1. **Simplicity** – No complex measurements. No hard-to-find ingredients. Just what you already have—elevated.

2. **Satiation over starvation** – Pink salt helps you feel full by calming the stress-hormone cycle that leads to emotional eating.

3. **Mineral replenishment** – Every recipe is a chance to support the root systems that handle cravings, energy, mood, and digestion.

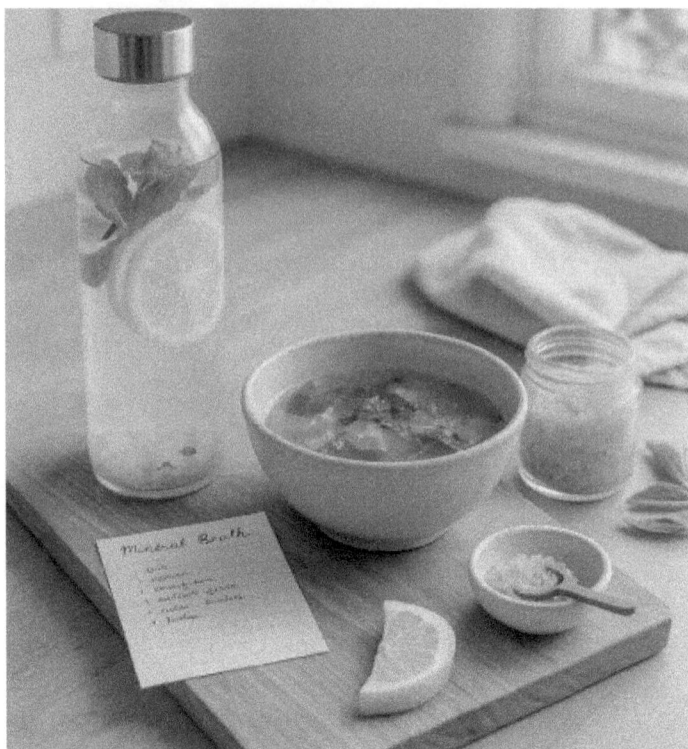

Salt isn't the villain. It's the forgotten healer. Taste, restore, and trust your cravings again.

CHAPTER 8

The Science Behind the Salt (Without the Jargon)

The truth behind your cravings, fatigue, and the pink salt that might just change everything.

Let's be honest—most "science chapters" are where wellness books go to die.

Charts, acronyms, and walls of text? No thanks.

This isn't that.

This chapter is your translation key—turning complex biology into simple truths. We're going to walk you through the actual science behind Himalayan pink salt and its effects on energy, hormones, hydration, and stress. No degrees required.

Just curiosity, clarity, and a pinch of wonder.

So... What Even Is Pink Salt?

Himalayan pink salt isn't just "pretty salt."

It's ancient. Primal. Over 250 million years old, actually harvested from fossilized seabeds buried deep beneath the Himalayan mountains of Pakistan. It's unrefined, hand-mined, and rich in trace minerals that give it that signature blush.

While table salt is stripped and bleached (think: 97% sodium chloride + additives), pink salt comes with a broad mineral spectrum that can include:

- Magnesium
- Potassium
- Calcium
- Iron
- Zinc
- Trace iodine (naturally occurring—not synthetic)

It's these **minerals**, not the pinkness, that make it matter.

Electrolytes 101 — The Simplified Version

You hear the word electrolytes and probably think of neon sports drinks. But here's the truth:

Electrolytes are minerals that conduct electricity in the body.

They carry signals between your brain and your cells, your muscles and your nerves. They are *essential* for hydration, digestion, heart rhythm, hormone production, and even mood stability.

The main electrolytes include:

- **Sodium** (yes, the "good" kind)
- **Potassium**
- **Magnesium**

- **Calcium**

- **Chloride**

And guess what?

Most people today are chronically deficient in several of these.

Not because they're unhealthy because they're *stressed, sweating, over-caffeinated,* and *under-mineralized*.

Which leads us to the real energy crisis...

The Hydration-Hormone-Fatigue Triangle

Here's a secret that could change your mornings forever:

Fatigue isn't always about sleep.

It's often about cellular dehydration and mineral loss.

Your hormones (like cortisol, insulin, estrogen, and thyroid messengers) rely on a well-hydrated, mineralized system. When you're depleted even just a little—your body can't fire on all cylinders. It conserves energy. It slows down metabolism. It triggers cravings to "wake you up."

So you reach for sugar. Or coffee. Or carbs.

But what your body is *really* asking for?

- Minerals.
- Salt.
- Nervous system safety.

Why Your Body Craves Salt Under Stress

Ever noticed how stress makes you want something salty?

That's not weakness—it's wisdom.

Your adrenal glands, which pump out stress hormones like cortisol and adrenaline, are **mineral-hungry**. When you're anxious, overwhelmed, or inflamed, they burn through sodium, potassium, and magnesium like wildfire.

"Salt cravings are often your body's request for *support*, not sabotage."

Low sodium can mimic depression.

Low magnesium can mimic anxiety.

Low potassium can mimic exhaustion.

No wonder everything feels *harder* when you're depleted.

The Myth of "Too Much Salt"

Let's bust a big one:

The **"low salt = healthy"** myth was built on shaky, outdated science.

Yes, processed table salt in junk food can raise blood

pressure in *sensitive individuals*. But that's not the same as hand-mined, mineral-rich salt used in a balanced, whole-food lifestyle.

In fact, new research shows that:

- **Too little salt** can raise stress hormones
- **Low sodium diets** may increase insulin resistance and fatigue
- **Natural salt** supports hydration, digestion, and hormonal resilience

And here's the best part:

When paired with proper hydration, lemon, and potassium-rich foods (like fruit and leafy greens**), pink salt becomes part of a mineral balancing act**, not a villain.

So... Does It Actually Work?

Thousands of women using this ritual would say yes.

But you don't have to take it on faith—this ritual is backed by:

- **Clinical data** on adrenal fatigue and sodium repletion

- **Peer-reviewed studies** on electrolyte balance and hormone function

- **Biological consensus** that cellular hydration requires sodium + potassium together

- **Nutritional evidence** linking low mineral intake with mood, metabolism, and fatigue disorders

Recap: What You Now Know

- Pink salt isn't trendy—it's ancient, mineral-rich, and metabolically supportive

- Minerals like magnesium and potassium are key to energy, hormone balance, and digestion
- Your fatigue may not be laziness—it may be low minerals and cellular stress
- Salt is not the enemy. Depletion is.
- You don't need to fear salt—you need to understand it

Let This Chapter Be Your Permission Slip

To stop fearing salt.

To stop blaming yourself for being tired.

To start drinking mineral water like it's sacred.

To reclaim energy by *replenishing*, not restricting.

Because real energy doesn't come from another shot of espresso.

It comes from restoring what your body has been begging for all along.

Salt. Sip. Rise. Repeat.

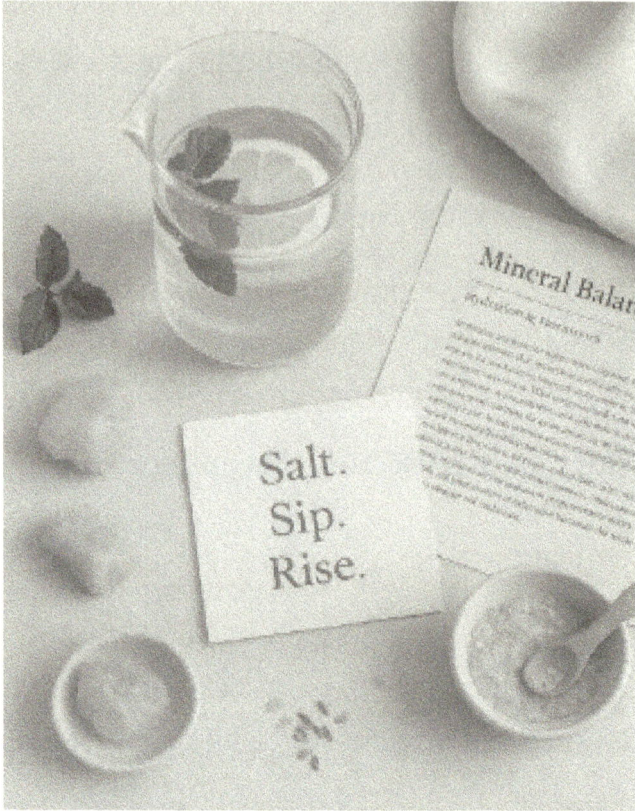

Fatigue isn't always about sleep. Sometimes it's about minerals. Fuel your cells, not just your calendar.

CHAPTER 9

Your New Normal: Staying Balanced Beyond the Reset

You didn't come this far to start over, you came this far to begin again and again, without fear. This chapter is your soft landing, your invitation to live the reset as a lifestyle, not a phase. Because balance isn't about being perfect, it's about knowing how to come home to yourself.

How to Maintain Your Glow (Without Obsession)

You've done the 21-day ritual. You've tasted clarity. You've felt what it means to wake up with lightness instead of heaviness, to crave nourishment instead of noise. Now what?

The truth is, the glow you've found isn't fragile. It doesn't require micromanaging your meals or fearing a "bad" food day. This chapter teaches you how to make your new normal feel intuitive. We'll help you anchor to what works without needing to obsess, track calories, or panic if you skip a tonic. You'll learn to shift your mindset from control to *connection*.

The rituals you've practiced aren't meant to trap you in rigidity—they're here to give you *rhythm*.

How to Bounce Back When Life Throws You Off

Travel, PMS, a tough work week, a last-minute takeout night—none of these are setbacks. They're part of life. The real power of the Pink Salt Ritual is not that it prevents chaos, but that it gives you a *way back*.

This chapter includes bounce-back protocols:

- The 24-Hour Salt Reset after a bloating or fatigue flare-up
- PMS Soothing Tonics to ground you during emotional waves
- Quick digestion resets after travel or heavy eating
- Fatigue rescue on days when burnout feels overwhelming

We'll walk you through how to soften instead of spiral, to return to your rituals instead of punish your body. You are not "starting over." You are continuing—wisely, kindly.

Mini Rituals for Real Life (Travel, PMS, Burnout Days)

You don't need to haul your whole pantry to feel supported.

Here's what you *can* bring:

- A travel sachet of pink salt and a slice of lemon in your carry-on
- A small dropper bottle of magnesium or trace minerals for hotel hydration
- A travel-size jar of salt scrub for grounding after long flights or draining meetings
- A PMS care card with your go-to calming blends, rituals, and affirmations

Your rituals can live in your purse, your journal, your intention. This chapter shows you how to build a toolkit of tiny, *mighty* resets that work when you're not at home or feeling off center.

The Salt Journal: How to Track

Energy, Cravings, and Mood

If willpower fades, rhythm carries you. And rhythm is born from awareness.

You'll learn how to keep a Salt Journal—not as a task list, but as a reflection space. It's not about perfection. It's about *pattern recognition*:

- What time of day do cravings spike?
- What rituals actually helped you feel better?
- When did you feel most energized? Most grounded?

We offer you simple daily prompts like:

- "What did I crave today?"
- "How did I support myself instead?"
- "One thing that made me feel calm…"

You'll come to see that your body speaks in patterns. The journal lets you listen.

Staying Light Without Willpower— Just Rhythm

Forget rigid rules. Forget punishment cycles. This chapter is your permission slip to live lightly, because you know how not because you're forcing yourself.

The salt rituals are now part of your nervous system, your kitchen, your mornings, your moon cycles. They're in your tea. In your bath. In your breath.

You now know how to:

- Start your day with minerals instead of caffeine
- Check in with your gut instead of your guilt
- Use flavor and intention as healing agents

Lightness becomes your baseline. Because you're not depriving you're *nourishing*.

This is your new normal: rooted, real, and replenished. Not

perfect. Just yours.

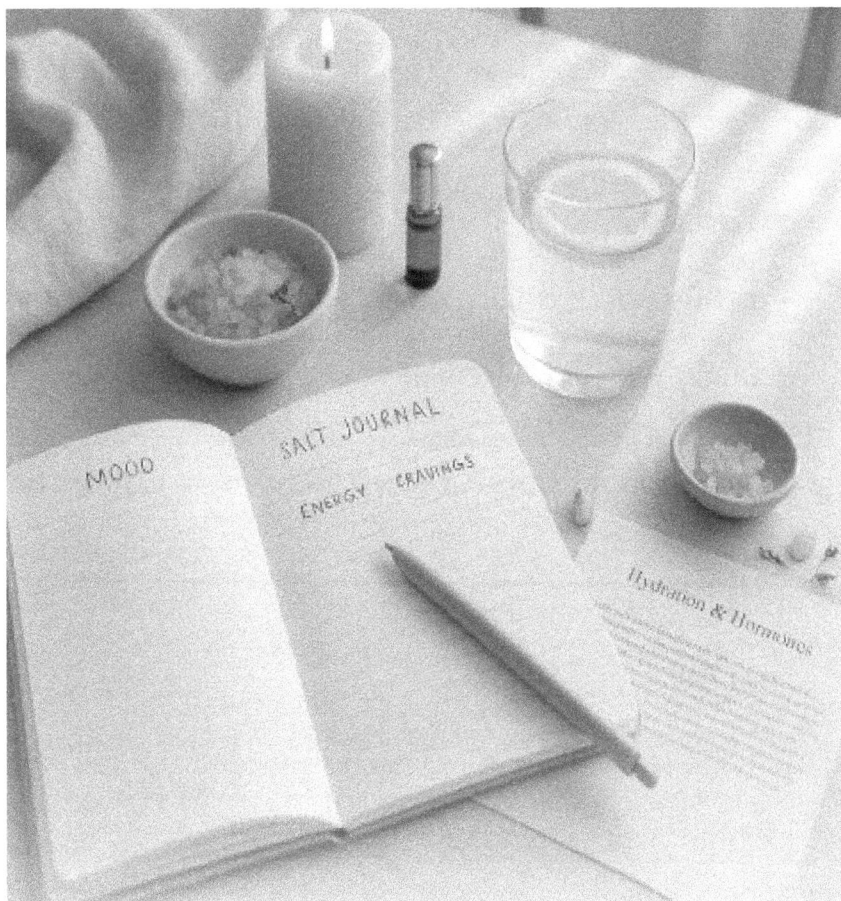

This isn't about sticking to a plan. It's about returning to yourself—again and again. That's the real reset.

What This Book Truly Delivers

This isn't another wellness trend dressed up in pink. It's a return to rhythm, to simplicity, to the kind of nourishment your body has been quietly asking for. Here are **the core themes** you'll experience as you turn the pages and as the ritual becomes your own:

✅ **Metabolism Support Through Hydration + Minerals**

No gimmicks. Just biology. When your cells are hydrated and mineral-fed, your metabolism starts to hum. Pink salt, paired with intentional hydration, unlocks the energy you've been trying to force through diets or supplements.

✅ **Hormone Harmony (Without Jargon or Fear)**

We don't weaponize hormones—we listen to them. This book explains the link between salt, stress, and sex hormones in a way that's calm, clear, and actionable. No fear. No shame. Just flow.

✅ Natural Energy and Stress Recovery

Your exhaustion isn't laziness—it's depletion. You'll learn how nervous system rituals and mineral repletion can gently bring your body out of fight-or-flight and into sustainable, calm energy. The kind that lasts beyond 3 p.m.

✅ Craving Control Using Nervous System Rituals

This is not about willpower. It's about safety. Your body craves sugar, starch, or caffeine when it feels stressed or unsatisfied. Through soothing rituals and mineral-rich nourishment, cravings naturally quiet. You'll stop fighting them—and start understanding them.

✅ Gut Support and Digestion Relief

Pink salt is a digestive ally. From bloating to sluggish metabolism, you'll discover how rituals and recipes in this book support your gut's ability to absorb, eliminate, and thrive. Expect flatter bellies and deeper comfort—not by force, but by flow.

✅ Empowerment Through Simplicity—Not Restriction

You won't find calorie counts or banned foods here. You'll find rhythms. Gentle, repeatable actions that build trust with your body—one salt sip, one mindful meal, one soothing soak at a time. This isn't about control. It's about collaboration with your biology.

✅ Human, Relatable Success Stories

You'll meet women who were once stuck, bloated, overwhelmed, or burnt out—just like you. And you'll see how simple rituals changed more than their jeans size. They regained peace, clarity, self-respect. Their stories will echo in you—and encourage your next step.

This book delivers results, yes. But more importantly, it delivers relationship with your body, your energy, your real needs. One mineral-rich moment at a time.

Acknowledgments

To the quiet mornings and the healing rituals that whispered, "*Start here.*"

To every woman who ever felt bloated, tired, confused, or defeated by her own body—I wrote this for you.

Thank you to my readers, friends, and early testers who believed in the power of pink salt before the world caught on. Your stories, feedback, and transformations gave this book its heartbeat.

www.ingramcontent.com/pod-product-compliance
Lightning Source LLC
Chambersburg PA
CBHW031130020426
42333CB00012B/316